PSYCHOSIS
A Figment of the Imagination ?

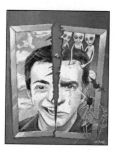

A
Martal Book
Publication

Front Cover illustrated
by
Valerie Peacock

Martal Book
Publications
This is a First Edition (April 2007)
ISBN 978-1-903256-36-7

FOREWORD

A factual, very personal account of an incident some years ago, which still affects my life to date, and of the difficult psychological problems originating from that time.

We all strive for a 'perfect' existence but that's never set in stone. When we change so dramatically before our very eyes, so too does our perception of others.

From seemingly having everything, to ending up with nothing, is tough to take.

The human mind is a complex thing and when even slightly unbalanced, can inexplicably alter our every positive trait.

'Follow your dreams.'

Nem0

CHAPTER ONE

For the first thirty-four years of my life, I couldn't complain. I had two adoring sisters, good, loyal, loving parents who taught me the rights and wrongs, gave me decent manners and the tools required to start out on my journey into this big daunting world.

There were some ups and downs along the way-we can't all be perfect. A couple of hormonally challenged teenage years perhaps, but nothing more than most families would have gone through.

I would describe myself as a fun-loving type of guy in those earlier periods of growing up and young adulthood - worked hard for a living, enjoyed a beer with plenty of laughs along the way, and made some trusted, dependable friends. I also had the classic roving eye for a pretty girl. But I was a single lad in those days, never did anyone any harm, just happy being me.

In those times as a youth and up to my early thirties, I had two main jobs. After leaving school at sixteen, a bricklaying job became available. I was an apprentice for four years, but alas it didn't blossom into fruition. In my case '1,000 a day brickie,' was never going to happen. The second type of employment was in stark contrast. I grafted for twelve years as a foundation worker, on the length and breadth of the railway networks, which gave me much more satisfaction and a lust for living.

Annual summer holidays abroad were a must, when a few pals and I would head for the sun. The Spanish or Greek islands were among our favourites. It just so happened that on one of these jolly jaunts I met my wife, or ex-wife as she is now. Funny, most people have the preconception that, with a holiday romance, when you return from the sun and sangria, it all fades into a distant hazy memory. In the past, I had been of the same persuasion. But this time was different.

I couldn't put my finger on it. In Greece, on a beautiful island, there she was. I felt an instant attraction and it seemed that the feelings were mutual. Just one tiny little problem was later to emerge - the fact that she was foreign and spoke very limited English. Moreover, I couldn't utter a word of her native tongue. It's at times like these that you wish you had learned the appropriate language at school. Even so we still spent a lot of time together. It felt like some-thing more this time, more than just being in 'the fling' category.

I suppose the sad feelings in the pit of the stomach on waving goodbye at the airport, almost certainly confirmed it. We managed to communicate somehow with hand gestures, head movements and a pal of hers was able to translate most of the English, which was invaluable. It was just enough for us to know how we felt about each other, and to hope-fully stay in touch.

I landed back home wiped out. Holidays often

seem to drain you like that, but unusually for me I felt strangely subdued. I knew I was missing the young lady to whom I had said "Cheerio" only three hours previously. The 'love' word springs to mind, which some men can find hard to admit to themselves, let alone say, but after just a couple of days, it was obvious to me that she was the one I hoped to spend the rest of my life with.

We kept in touch regularly, by phone, or writing letters to one another, which then led on to her coming over to see me, and vice-versa. Things were getting pretty intense now, in a short space of time. We had big decisions to make.

I decided that I would down tools, so to speak, and move to be with her. It was risky giving up a job that had served me well for so many years, and leaving behind family and friends. Even so, I still thought it was worth trying. Thinking back on the first time she stayed at my parent's home, she was already missing her cat and feeling homesick, so there seemed little chance of her upping sticks and moving from her country - that would have been a bit cruel. So, on that basis, I believe I made the right choice.

So, from our initial meeting in September to the following March, in only six months, we'd done it. Reunited, living together, a couple. Foolish? Not thought out? Maybe, but I always think you have to follow your heart. Do what is right for the best at that time. Up until now, even though circumstances have changed me so much, I have never once regretted the path I took, and would never consider it to be a mistake.

Okay, I may not be that happy-go-lucky young man that I was in my prime, and may seem totally unrecognisable now, in how I perceive myself, but fate can, at any stage, play a fickle hand to absolutely anybody. There are no set rules. Life can be soul destroying. If I had not grasped the nettle and gone for it, I would always have been left wondering, "What if....?"

The experience of relocating brings up many difficulties and emotions. I believe that most folk who move abroad would be lying if they didn't admit to feeling some home-sickness and isolation at first. We can all get teething troubles whilst trying to adapt or settle in. I can remember early on, many instances of getting things totally wrong, almost daily. Not picking up the right produce in the supermarket, passing a hammer instead of a screwdriver at work. Every little detail you can imagine, I was absolutely way out on.

It's lovely that we have all these islands and continents around the globe. But speaking the language, that's another matter. No one tells you that the locals haven't the time to wait for an Englishman, frantically flicking through a dictionary, or punching a pocket translator, to ask them a question. Even in the faint hope of getting some kind of reply, the answer would have still been mis-interpreted. This can leave you feeling both frustrated and inadequate. Although the early days were particularly tricky, I did see light at the end of the tunnel. Most people appreciate and applaud someone who makes a conscious effort to fit in.

The first year of my new adventure was finally panning out nicely. I managed now to get regular income rather than 'bits and bobs' in part-time situations, a real achievement for me. At last I was moving in the right direction and paydays were okay too. The natural progression now was for my girlfriend to become my fiancée. I cannot praise her family enough for the help and kindness they showed me, ferrying me round to interviews, frequent meals together on a weekend, always welcoming. I truly felt accepted by them all, which was now just as well because that once-in-a-lifetime moment had arrived, sitting in our cramped but practical one bed-roomed flat with the pet cat and the in-laws around the coffee table.

We announced our intentions to officially become an item and marry. I think they were pleased, judging from the firm handshakes, hugs and smiles being dished out. Or maybe it was just the plentiful amounts of beer and wine suddenly hitting the mark, but I doubt that somehow.

Let's not bore you too much with the pre-nuptials and wedding details. They were pretty much run of the mill, in the fact that it was held in a registry office. In my case with an interpreter, which helped. Especially knowing when to say, "I do," at the right time! The rings were exchanged and a party with family and friends ensued, with boogieing, some nifty, and some not-so-nifty, dance moves on display. A good time was had by all.

On leaving the celebrations before the end, as newlyweds often do, we got back to our newer flat to be greeted by balloons every-where. Someone had obviously sneaked the keys earlier, been in and bedecked much of the living room and bedroom with them. Not the best of ideas on our part though, to start popping them at midnight or one o`clock in the morning. I am sure the neighbours were not impressed. You hear of a lot worse pranks that people have had played on them on occasions like these, so I suppose balloons may seem fairly tame in comparison. Even so it was nice to know that someone took the trouble, if a little unexpected.

Waking up as Mr and Mrs, I am sure many couples would agree, is a wonderful feeling. It finally seemed to add more purpose and meaning to my life - the icing on the cake. We didn't plan to have children any time soon. Our ideal plan was to fit it in when the time felt right, but getting some savings together would be our first priority. Being relatively young, we had lots of years ahead before we needed to even contemplate the patter of tiny feet.

I do, however, recall one episode about seven or eight months into our marriage when this could have been a distinct possibility. In our love-life my wife took the contraceptive pill, but they sometimes didn't agree with her. She would often get tummy upsets and discomfort, so for a healthier balance tried different tablet types. On this occasion she was more than three weeks out with the menstrual cycle, and we even bought a home tester gadget, thinking that a pregnancy could unexpectedly be upon us. We talked the whole scenario through, such as the pros and cons of having a child at this stage, and whether the two of us could cope with such a huge responsibility. Needless to say it was a question we didn't have to answer. Slowly her stomach subsided, her body clock returned to normal, and a negative line showed up on the pregnancy kit. Who knows what may have happened in my life had the situation been the reverse.

CHAPTER TWO

I sometimes wonder if anyone can truthfully say they have always had the perfect partnership. I can only stand and admire those who honestly answer "Yes". Surely spats and tiffs are commonplace? Perhaps a few jealousies and insecurities crept in early on with us, but we managed to iron most of them out. However, just when I thought everything was on an even keel, a kick in the stomach was about to be administered. Could it have been the unsociable shift patterns I worked that played a part? Who knows. But it gave my wife way too much time on her hands, especially in the evenings, when she would take it upon herself to socialize with colleagues more often than usual. We were almost like passing ships at one point. I had my quiet suspicions that she may have been enjoying herself a little too much. Mixing with single friends can have a tendency to suck you in and I don't think much persuasion was needed on her part.

I remember the occasion vividly. After a rare night in together for once, the morning dawned and I felt great. We were decorating at this stage, as the bedroom and hallway needed papering and sprucing up. Whilst I agreeably carried on, she was off out for another sun-tanning session. Nothing new there! I loved exercise, whilst getting brown and having manicures was her thing. After kissing goodbye at the door I plodded on laying the lino down and what an un-forgiving task that was! A jigsaw puzzle would have been easier to fathom out. (D.I.Y. expert would never be written on my CV). It didn't look too bad actually. A smart move on my part though, keeping all the wrong cuts strategically hidden as you walked in.

Upon her arrival back late that afternoon, I showed the now newly laid masterpiece, (or not, in my case). She just about acknowledged it, which was nice, considering I had been snipping away all day. There was definitely an atmosphere around. I knew she'd had a couple of drinks by her demeanour - being giddy and giggly gave it away and the spearmint chewing gum did nothing to hide the vapours. I knew intuitively that something was amiss and didn't seem right. I found out soon enough.

Putting the greasy plates in the dishwasher was the last job to do. On sitting down I asked her what was up and if I had done any thing to upset her. It seemed that was just the cue she needed, brazenly telling me, "It's over." She wanted us to split up as she had feelings for another man. In that moment I reeled with shock and disbelief, surely it had not boiled down to this? I never saw it coming. How could she possibly proclaim to have affections for somebody else? I don't know what sort of a reaction she was hoping for. Shouts and screams, or slaps? That's not my way, even though it may have seemed to be deserved. All I could manage was question after question. Why? How long? There were no genuine replies forthcoming. The only crumb of comfort I could take, if any, was that she hadn't actually slept with him yet. I did believe her. Lying at this stage wouldn't have done any good. The worst part for me was her yearning and desire for another male. Wasn't I enough? It took me long into the night to make some kind of sense of it all. You could have stuck up a brick-wall in between us.

The next morning I tried everything I could to persuade her to give it another shot, short of begging on my hands and knees, but even that wouldn't have been good enough. The long stony silences followed, accompanied by a big dark cloud of uncertainty. I was walking on eggshells most days, praying that the words I did say to her were justified, otherwise there was a good chance that ranting and ridicule would be slung back in my direction. It made me feel like the potential marriage breaker here. I'd get up not knowing what kind of mood she was in and wondering if the suitcases had already been packed.

My wife would have been quite happy to ship me off back to England, sweep everything under the carpet, restart her life and pretend I never existed. Well, it wasn't going to happen. She was extremely surprised and no doubt disappointed when I decided to stick with it, especially with work, where I was progressing very well and now firmly established. Add to that my parents not being very pleased with her shenanigans and the in-laws near enough disowning her. She found that her once calculating, cold exterior guise was crumbling. Faced with this onslaught a truce became necessary.

Little by little the spark did re-ignite, we were interacting once again and making another go of it. I wasn't always sure first off if she was being genuine, or just flattering to deceive. Many a time I felt like smashing our happy wedding photo and replacing it with a blank piece of card, but she advised against this, said our love was unconditional and such a painful experience would never happen again. Thankfully it didn't. We were now re-established as the joyful adoring couple.

Because everything was running smoothly and contentedly once more, we needed a treat to acknowledge the fact. On putting our heads together, the idea of this once-in-a-lifetime exotic holiday popped out from the brochure we scanned. We hadn't had any kind of honeymoon as such, so what better way to have a double celebration and forget about past misdemeanours? There were two choices originally but after some deliberation we plumped for 'The One!' An idyllic tropical island that had clear blue waters fringed with lush, white sandy beaches, red hot sun and the best scenic views imaginable. Truly heaven sent. The flight would be ten hours or more, a long way, but sore posteriors wouldn't be a problem for us, knowing what delights this oasis by the Indian Ocean had to offer. We booked up immediately. It would be costly, more than your average run-of-the-mill package deal, but it seemed so perfect for us, that turning down this opportunity wasn't an option.

On boarding the aeroplane that July we en-
countered some small amounts of turbulence
when passing through different air currents
and climates, but nothing drastic. On a long
haul journey like this you're bound to hit the
odd wobble or two. So with our stomachs
intact and no sick bags needed we dis-
embarked, drained but cheerful.

The initial few hours after landing were spent
sorting out the accommodation and getting a
rough idea where all the amenities were
situated. It was a place that was as good as it
said in the book, if not more so. Our swish
upmarket beach hut was almost in touching
distance of the wonderful coastline, and
everything top notch. Apart from one small
niggle or observation. We would sometimes
find the occasional unwanted house -guest
(not contributing any rent!) I don't mean a
spider, or an ugly cockroach. No! This was
somewhat bigger on its pins. A lizard (gecko)
had decided to move in with us, in fact more

than one.

The thatch-like roofing and cupboard areas seemed quite popular for these creatures to have a poke around. I first noticed them when I nonchalantly looked towards the ceiling whilst relaxing on our bed, and almost did a double take, seeing this green thing with legs, creeping amongst the rafters. It was reassuring to know that they didn't bite and were extremely common around these parts. We did get used to them in a fashion though I'm sure the both of us slept with one eye open.

The first week of this sixteen-day adventure passed in a hurry. Many a lazy afternoon was had by the sea and lovely meals were eaten restaurant- style, or out on our plush patio area. We did plenty of touring as well, spying very large tortoises, crocodiles, monkeys, butterflies and various species of colourful birds in enclosures. Not forgetting the temples, beautiful flowers and breathtaking sights of green velvet and golden-yellow plateaux all around. We used a personal chauffeur for these excursions (a taxi really, but it had that same feel,) which always meant we got knowledgeable running commentaries whilst travelling to points of interest; a better way to explore for my money, because it always strikes me that when you use pre-organised coach trips, you are often crammed in like sardines and then guided around en masse. It doesn't quite have that same romantic ambience as exploring together as a couple.

Alas! From this point onwards my own down-ward spiral would begin. From being such a captivating awe-inspiring dream, our holiday would now become unbearable and problem-strewn. I'll explain.

From the eighth day forward, a new crop of holidaymakers descended on the resort, interchanging with people returning back home, unfortunately for me bringing in a few clusters of single lads. Nothing wrong with that in principle; I could recall being young, free and single myself not so long ago, which meant plenty of hard partying to be done, particularly on 18-30 Club holidays, incorporating frolics and general mayhem. But this was hardly Ibiza, or Gran Canaria, where there would have been hordes of single females. Our retreat predominately appealed to the lovey-dovey twosome, or already attached type folk.

Nothing too sinister transpired; a few wolf whistles were heard and admiring glances given (not for me I should add!) but directed almost certainly towards my wife, who admittedly was attractive as well as compatible; a real catch in my eyes. However, leading on from that, certain individuals would, blatantly, every morning, strategically plonk their towels on the sand, only a few metres below our abode. I didn`t really understand why they would continuously keep that same spot, especially on a wide open beach, where one would have been spoilt for choice to sunbathe and swim. They always had the knack of being in view and, on more than a few occasions, leering suggestively at my partner. Our way to counteract this was by going shopping, having long strolls near the waters edge and taking moonlight dips.

It had little effect in the grand scheme of things. Many a time, while we were getting ready for an evening meal or just catnapping, these youths would not be far away. Lack of single lasses must have played a part; not a good mix with male testosterone, but hardly my problem. They might just as well have been statues or stuck in cement, such was the lack of movement shown during those last days of our stay.

I was getting angry, frustrated and unnerved by this display. It wouldn't have been so bad had they varied their routine sometimes, instead of constantly appearing near us, or in our faces. Ordinarily I would have confronted these idiots or had a quiet word and defused a potential incident, (fighting for me is always the very last option) as it was causing unnecessary friction, but nobody wants aggravation, even less so on a honeymoon island, where you would hope to rise above stresses and petty squabbles. As I'm a law-abiding citizen, I wouldn't have relished the idea of maybe spending time stuck in some cold cell, out in the middle of nowhere, through somebody else's actions. Most countries won't stand for any nonsense, but troublemakers can reach even the most serene of locations and, when tanked up on bellyfuls of beer, have no regard for rationality or reasoning. We even informed night security, such was the extent of the intrusive behaviour, and we felt that it messed up our great getaway irrevocably. Sadly, this left me feeling relieved that our outward trek home was drawing nearer. I would then be back on familiar soil, free from this bewildering madness.

CHAPTER THREE

Madness. The word itself conjures up all kinds of definitions, and some people might jest about it, telling comical anecdotes, while others find it rather more serious and often unexplainable. Perhaps being confused or being unsure in oneself is sometimes a more accurate diagnosis. I was certainly going to become confused, (that's an understatement!) if nothing else, by the time we were re-acquainted with our cat, flat, and my comfy armchair. There was I thinking a few unruly fools from that sun-kissed isle had been problematic; well I was in for a more compounding, traumatic shock.

The return journey on the jumbo jet began pleasantly enough. We both found our seats, plugged in stereo music headphones, then up and away she soared. About an hour or so into the flight nature called; I tried holding it in for as long as possible, because aeroplane lavatories are not the biggest or most comfortable of spaces to inhabit. When poodling back down the aisle on finishing my ablutions, I happened by chance and in quite an innocent fashion to make eye contact with three individuals, two male and one female, who were sitting near us, some four rows back.

They didn't exactly exchange what you would call amiable glances with me, but instead, cold, piercing, steely stares, from all three of them simultaneously. I tried not dwelling on the matter, and thought perhaps their holiday had turned out naff too. But after this initial eyeballing, at intervals, verbal heckling became audible, to me anyway, if nobody else, in a tone that was hateful and vicious in content. The expletives "Bastard," "Pr---," "Arse----," and a word rhyming with anchor were complimentary, compared to some uttered! I knew for certain that this was aimed towards me, and other more flattering remarks towards my wife. "Pretty," correct. "Fair haired," correct. "Foreign," correct.

"Sat by the window," also correct. They used these subject themes, with snide innuendo, in a running commentary, right up until we landed on terra firma.

My suspicions were confirmed further by our brief stop for refuelling, when the identical trio, sure as eggs, circulated stealthily round about us in the waiting area. Call it instinct or foresight, I just knew these people were bad apples and would become my worst nightmare.

You may ponder how, during this entire hullabaloo, the Mrs was coping. One must state, "Surprisingly well," in fact, calmness personified. She didn't however know the English dialect and accents so intimately as I did, so she was unaware how what I had witnessed had culminated in this spiteful, festering, smog-heavy atmosphere. It was totally uncomfortable and unsettling for me. A situation arising completely out of the blue, which I felt I couldn't control or stop.

The last leg of our flight drew to a close and with the runway at long last emerging into focus we prepared to touch down. Travelling drags out considerably when one feels pressured or overpowered by tension and I spoke tersely to my wife, on alighting from our seats, imploring "Let's not hang about, just grab the luggage as quickly as possible, hail a cab and get home". She looked at me curiously but I wasn't in any mood for small talk or explanations, hoping that, eventually, when my key unlocked our front door, my life could return to some sort of normality.

Teacup nestled in one hand, duty-free cigarette clasped in the other, I dared to believe that this seemingly endless mini crisis could be over. It was strangely ironic that sitting there in the living room brought me more euphoria than those last days of our doom- filled holiday. We were obviously at this point overwhelmingly jetlagged from our weary travels, so, after nipping to the local store for some essentials, bed and slumber sounded a good idea.

I was unable to sleep so I thought it best to have another brew in the kitchen, rather than disturb my beloved, who was snoring merrily away. Lucky her! Oblivious of any problems, I took my next sip. Suddenly, to my absolute astonishment, familiar voices came into range, which I thought I had heard for the last time, not directly outside our property but certainly within earshot. (Remember that this was at the height of summer, so our windows were ajar.) You cannot imagine how utterly disconcerted and confused I felt. I was dumb-struck. Could it possibly have transpired that those people, the individuals from the aircraft, were in our midst, on our street, on our estate? Perhaps I had got my wires crossed, needed extra shut-eye, wasn't fully alert? Deep down I knew that no amount of kip or berating myself could persuade me otherwise. I was a level headed, clear-thinking young man, the same as any other person, and I knew what I had heard.

Outrageously far-fetched and in-comprehensible events do occur in life, thankfully few and far between. Never-the-less, these things can happen to anybody in an unlucky minority of cases, as I began to realise. The days following this in our flat didn't get much easier, and I often mused whether I was delusional, as a sense of cracking up was gradually creeping over me. Consider momentarily the emotion of extreme envy, obsessive human beings who will stop at nothing to attain a goal. They're crafty, devoid of all normal feelings, sly, and want everything you've got which they haven't. As dramatic as this reads, this was my predicament.

From being formerly a fairly athletic, strong guy, I was to become an eight and a half stone or less, shuffling, shambling, weakened wreck. During so many nights of cold sweats and insomnia, too numerous to calculate, I couldn't switch off. My ears were now like radio antennae, forever listening out, picking up any little rustles or murmurings, (having paper-thin walls didn't help my cause). It got to a stage where I would shut the curtains by daylight and sit in different corners of our rooms, two fingers firmly plugged in my lugholes, trying desperately for some peace and quiet, which never came, amidst an onslaught of belittling degradation. A fortnight or more later, they still hadn't gone. One of the trio in particular despised me intensely, such were his stalker-type characteristics on display, which I felt and breathed every waking minute.

Even to this point in my life I've always honestly believed that he harboured insane jealousy towards me, for having an alluring wife. He clearly thought she could have chosen much more wisely. To him I was no better than dirt on a shoe or dregs of some used wine bottle, (what a lovely view of me he had .... not!!).

Make-believe and fantasies I generally don't do, and there were two more decisive happenings, which one hundred percent re-confirmed my suspicions and removed any lingering doubts I may originally have had.

The first oddity centred around our communal laundry enclosure, where paying tenants, including us, could hang up or air wet clothing. On the day in question, whilst pegging out a full basket load, I'd noticed an entrance door was slightly open, which was standard procedure when doing this task. Unbelievably for me, yet again prominent regional English twangs materialised and I don't mean in muffled, low tones. This became coherent, close, too close for comfort and still its vocabulary and intent aimed specifically at me.

I'd completely crumbled by now, my mind shot to pieces, no longer having any mental or physical capabilities for proper functioning. I couldn't even confront these seemingly desperate tormentors, such was the grip they held over me, and the damaging effect they now had, (how pathetic is that?)

With the second incident things became even more vivid and eerie. It concerned our weekly supermarket shop, which I would regularly do with my mother in-law. She had the car and could drive, plus we'd have a good old chinwag. Alas, due to these unforeseen provocations my nattering days were to be effectively over. We filled up our trolleys and proceeded towards the checkouts. Trying to be inconspicuous, I looked back at my ever-increasing queue, and unerringly spotted those same three characters. Clear as crystal, almost within spitting distance, each with the same demeanour, the same physique, and the same language. I thought I had spied them moments earlier, pretending to choose items of food from the shelves.

There was no further proof now needed for me. This could not be normal behaviour surely, could it? Just think, starting from on board an aeroplane, escalating into finding ones abode, loitering around for nigh on three weeks and continually tracking my every footstep. It seemed like some kind of sick joke. Unfortunately for me I was living this.

I'd gone blank after leaving the store, head spinning, legs feeling like lead. My mum in-law even suggested waiting for the three-some outside, but it was, sadly, too little, too late for me now. The spirit and fight I may have shown a couple of months prior had evaporated; I had no energy. Uncontrollable panic struck. I'd heard and seen enough of this group to last an eternity. It sent shivers down my spine to even contemplate re-confirming their existence, so we drove off.

The impact of this entire chilling episode had left its mark. I began acting in a strangely erratic way, completely out of character. For example, writing down on lined paper detailed descriptions of these aggressors, showing them to my beloved and then promptly but delicately placing them inside a drawer for safe keeping, just on the off chance that something sinister should occur. At other times, when lying down, (snoozing was now impossible) I'd hide a blunt metal object under the pillow, and had also taken to sitting transfixed by my wife's side of the bed, with an old starting pistol in hand, (I didn't and wouldn't use or fire one, I hasten to add!). At least, if the door had suddenly burst open, it may have seemed that I was prepared. I'd be kidding myself if I thought that being paralysed by this constant surmounting fear meant being prepared. It was small compensation, when morning came, to realise that at least I had survived another day.

From here on in there were no more good times or happy events. My whole persona was irreversibly turned upside down. Everybody, especially my family, were extremely concerned and worried about me, so much so that my own mother flew over twice. I must have had the resemblance of a skeleton when she first clapped eyes on me. I had become mere skin and bone. Her once healthy boy was in a real state. Unfortunately, the sounds, voices, people I'd heard or seen couldn't be corroborated by my mum, so with no clear cut evidence for her to substantiate this earnest account of mine, how would I ever be believed?

The perpetrators knew when to be silent and when to talk by now. I would even, in theatrical fashion, put drinking glasses on our floorboards, tentatively listening to the flat below for signs or indications of audible mutterings and almost always getting that same unwanted answer, "YES", or was it only my ears deceiving me?

Perhaps inevitably my work began to suffer very badly. I managed to last out seven days (surprisingly) from our initial return from holiday, but so feeble had my strength become and so deeply did I feel pursued, that the sick leave, which the firm suggested, seemed the only option.

CHAPTER FOUR

A man having a nervous breakdown? I didn't like to admit it, but I had to face the fact that something was definitely wrong with me. As much as I'd fought against accepting any help, continuous badgering from my wife and two mothers brought the inevitable outcome. A discussion with the local consultant was deemed necessary, though somewhat begrudgingly agreed by me. How I made it to his waiting room and office I'll never know, as it was, for me, like a man striving to conquer Everest - extremely risky! Any outside activities had become beyond impossible. I was forever nervy, on edge and un-relaxed, with feelings of discomfort about everything.

The doctor gave his summing up after hearing the relevant information, data and subjective theories. Medical people may be open-minded or impartial but at this point he must have concluded that he was dealing with some off beat ramblings, so unrealistic that they held no truth, but pure, contrived fiction. I will always beg to differ. Let's just say the prognosis didn't fill one with joy. The name, 'PSYCHOSIS'. Definition: A severe mental derangement, especially when resulting in delusions and loss of contact with external reality. Fleetingly past his lips came a word and its meaning that was hard to accept. Couldn't they be wrong for once in their lives? Mis-read the script perhaps? Perhaps I was one of a select few who had just been delivered a bad hand?

My fate had now been signed and sealed, an uncertain future hanging precariously on the coat tails of the medical profession. Would my life ever revert to those almost forgotten heady days? My first move towards the possibility of stability came via a week of intensive medication (tablets) recommended by the doctor. I was to finish this cocktail of potent pills, in varying quantities and types, at home in the flat. My mother, bless her, oversaw everything. She administered the treatments when required, cooked and cleaned, and was a real rock for me, as I wasn't allowed to be left alone. Some flicker of hope emerged initially but, alas, it didn't last. No sooner had my mother thought things were on an upward curve and she could return to Britain, when once again the walls came tumbling down.

I'd finished the required course of treatment, contentedly musing that I was fixed, cured, and my doctor had, at an earlier meeting, declared, "No further action will be needed." He lied! Desperate foot stamping and wrangling proved futile on my part. His decision was final. Nothing I said could persuade him otherwise. This meant only one outcome; my transferral into a place so severely stigmatised and falsely vilified that it brought goose pimples to my skin.

My recollection of the classic movie 'One Flew Over the Cuckoo's Nest,' supplied me with images of similarities to myself. Psychiatric placement! Those establishments are for mad, loony lowlifes aren't they? After all that's what the general public's perception seems to be. Funny how, ordinarily, you would need a straight jacket to stop me kicking and screaming on entering such a forbidding building, but, because of my ever worsening fragile state of mind I was merely mouse-like, subdued, totally oblivious. In other circumstances the transferral would have had the appearance of some family day out, a car filled with relatives, my case neatly packed, only this was to be no picnic or ice-cream licking occasion. My new residence blinked on the horizon. Okay, it didn't look old or shabby, in fact just the opposite. Beautiful flowered gardens and ponds arranged around modern buildings. No barbed wire or heavy pad-locked gates, in fact it seemed as though you could come and go as you pleased. Escape appeared to be easy-peasy.

I sat by the foyer of my allocated treatment ward, mother in-law one side, and the wife the other, not uttering a single word, just staring wide eyed into space, wrapped up within my own isolated, jumbled up world where no-one else was allowed. I noticed on arrival an in-patient rocking vigorously on a chair, horseman like. Others passed by either very quickly or the complete opposite, slow, lethargic, snail-paced. Which type would I morph into I wondered? We said our good-byes, they'd keep in touch, (loved ones) see me daily if possible. All I knew was that I didn't want to be there. I wish I'd turned right around and walked straight back out.

Freedom seemed a far-flung memory. It took me fully three weeks to convince myself that my torturers had finally crawled back into their own non-existent lives, (my view) having already ruined mine. They got what they wanted didn't they, but the aftermath was inconceivable. I now felt pre-judged; I despised my appearance, hated the thought of anyone noticing me and, sadly, also felt a sense of complete social detachment.

I'd taken some time settling into the regime of

the hospital and every day brought similarly monotonous tasks. There were indoor sports, exercises to take part in, long walks around the grounds, mini bus trips and rest periods. All well and good when in peak condition, but so diverse was our range of problems and difficulties that appreciating these activities proved difficult. Early mornings were the hardest times, when we patients had to group together in semi-circular fashion, then expound with enlightenment on how we felt and what our aspirations might be. This was rather strange considering that there seemed little or no hope in most cases, at that early stage. I also found that my English, as well as my newly adopted language, had almost completely eradicated itself from my memory. If I did communicate it would only consist of short, gruff sentences in low monotone drawls. I did not want to be seen or heard for heavens sake! How could interacting help? It seemed only to heighten my paranoid inadequacies.

There was one friendly lad of Middle Eastern

descent who I gelled with. He forever poured words of wisdom on me and kept my dwindling spirits up by quoting meaningful extracts from God-centred books, almost putting his own troubles aside for my needs. He'll never know how truly grateful I was. In order to just wake up and get by every day in such an intense environment, one requires some form of guidance.

Pills were regularly dished out like 'Smarties' among us. At certain times I ingested nine different sorts in a sitting, including anti-psychotics, anti- depressants, tranquillisers and other tablets to counteract side effects! I wondered why I was taking so many. Not surprising then that I turned zombie-like, disorientated and with disconcerting bodily shakes, especially in my hands. Holding a cup of water or an item of cutlery still, without twitching, became humiliating and I spilt more food down my clothes than I managed to spoon-feed into my mouth. I suppose the medics were trying to realign my brain functions and balance out or suppress irrational signals. Well, they certainly didn't hold back on the drugs cabinet! It wasn't exclusively tablets though.

The mini-van was used for three of us once, for a drive to some location where I presumed experts wished to delve further into our minds. A big long rotating machine, which I later discovered was an M.R.I scanner, greeted me, accompanied by small computer-type monitoring screens dotted about an examination room. My whole body was placed onto the waiting contraption, with just the top half to be encased. It had the appearance of some weird time machine. Pity I couldn't be instantly transported back to happier carefree years. Its procedure didn't last long but I'd no idea what the results or findings were. Standard practice presumably.

There arose one other occasion when a bizarre alternative therapy was incorporated into my treatment plan. In this instance a skullcap, (not your fancy swimming-pool hair accompaniment,) sprouting protruding wires was strategically positioned upon my head. It didn't hurt but looked rather silly. Okay for a fancy-dress ball I guess, but presumably the purpose of it was to elicit responses of some form or other, as its operator fired random questions at me. Beeping noises would also play intermittently and melodically.

My stay with the institution lasted roughly three weeks, but I couldn't honestly say I'd progressed at all; in truth I probably exited a whole lot worse. Talking on the telephone to anybody, including my mother, was increasingly awful; I became incoherent, I whispered, and was not forthcoming with any reasonable sense whatsoever. I loathed the idea of people listening or acknowledging my voice. My mother had obviously decided enough was enough. She returned swiftly and gave the hospital entourage a few stern words about their holding back on translations, therefore not enabling me to fully interpret their procedures.

My poor state was cause for concern, so yet another meeting/get-together happened. Going home to England seemed feasible, but would also highlight a very big dilemma. How could I choose between this supposedly new beginning with my wife and in-laws, or Blighty? It was a decision only I could make. At that particular time the nurses and drugs had a totally mesmerising grip over me, so what sort of existence could I hope to achieve when I wasn't even in control of my own destiny? To go back to my roots would seem as though I'd failed somehow. I couldn't hack life in another country. I was a dead loss and had had work and foreign family prospects cruelly stolen from me. You could say I didn't have much sparkle left!

I am realistic though; you cannot put a price on health. If one lacks that, or peace of mind, life will always be a monumental struggle. I made my impossible decision and knew that I must get away from the scenes and surroundings of these nightmares, trusting that English care and support might perhaps alter things.

Waving goodbye to my wife wasn't easy. I often ponder in retrospect on what she also went through; a complete shock no doubt, seeing my character transformation and listlessness. The husband I once aspired to be was melting like a candle before her very eyes, my sanity and body dripping, ebbing towards an uncertain outcome. There seemed little that she could do or say. We (mother and I) landed on home turf after a difficult angst-filled flight, my mind still awash with medication, spinning with fast then slow shifts into light-headedness. I'd managed to navigate and stumble my way back into my former home a shadow of my true self, no bunting or fanfares, no celebrations or joyous welcoming, just deep inane feelings of emptiness.

My spirits were at an all-time low and I'd taken to lying in bed for obscenely long hours with sheets covering my head, as it felt like escape or respite. It acted only as a smoke screen. My now scruffy, unshaven, greasy-haired appearance matched this ugly, overweight body and bloated features. I didn't bother with mirrors any more. Why would I want to look at me? Family members rallied and tried their utmost to 'snap me out of it, pull myself together' but I was far beyond that.

Psychiatrists came and went; some good and some not so good. The dreaded tablets still profoundly impaired my judgement, although, thank God, they were eventually reduced in strength. I couldn't do anything because of the social anxiety, panic episodes and severe depression creeping over me. It became so debilitating that lifts to and from appointments were needed. I'd attempted public transport limitedly until a bad turn occurred, and ever since that occasion I have never been able to sit on a bus or even stand in the queue. Lapses of concentration occurred frequently, meaning that my mother had to fill in important paperwork.

Every passing second of those early days washed straight over me, as I was totally unresponsive to anything or anyone. My wife visited twice but I hardly registered the fact, wasn't great company if truth be told. I couldn't go anywhere let alone entertain. Strange thoughts still dominated my life, but at least inside my four walls I had an iota of calmness. Sensations of isolation and alienation were commonplace for me now; I even felt like a stranger in our family abode. How absurd is that?

There was no way of changing my mindset or rationalising my illogical notions. Existing in this fashion meant something had to give and it did. The hammer blow came after seeing my wife one last time and then receiving a phone call from her a month or so later. Our marriage was over, finished, as simple as that; it became especially hard to contemplate in my vulnerable state of mind. Maybe she couldn't handle the prospect of my never fully recovering? Perhaps a clean break was her motive, but it's something I'll be unlikely ever to know or totally comprehend. I would like to think that, if the shoe had been on the other foot, I'd have stuck by her and nursed her through. It seemed our marriage vows of 'In sickness and in health' counted for nothing. Had I now become a burden, an obstacle blocking her path? For whatever puzzling reason the matter was irretrievable, no re-conciliation. We've never spoken since but, rather poignantly, her parents still keep in contact, and show me empathy and concern, traits that must have by-passed my now-separated wife.

I've mellowed over these years and don't blame her at all for my own downfall or mis-givings. If circumstances were different, then maybe one's life would be too. I'm just so relieved that children didn't enter into the equation. My wife's shocking announcement none the less had a massive impact. I was extremely distraught, indeed almost inconsolable, my mind bubbling with dark thoughts of utter despair. There surfaced only one drastic step to take. The ultimate sin or a cry for help?

CHAPTER FIVE

Had I really sunk so deep that death, ending it all, seemed my only salvation? Stuck in no-mans-land with walls squeezing up tight, teetering on a precipice, the idea to me at that moment didn't seem foolhardy or unrealistic. I'd part planned it anyway, cunningly, secretly stocking up with Anadin, waiting for an opening, a chance when nobody was home.

This chance occurred one particular evening whilst my folks were out till late socialising. It was a perfect opportunity, and I had managed to conceal from them my inner hopelessness. However, it didn't quite work out how I'd imagined. I swallowed thirty pills all told, some singly, others five at a time, wondering after tablet number four if I was doing the right thing here. I decided it was too late now, so I would continue. When all the Anadins were finally consumed and washed down, groggy, nauseous sensations quickly developed. I lay on the double bed with my head numb and my stomach churning like a cement mixer, and then shut my eyes …. Nothing happened. Where were the bright guiding lights, pearly gates, heaven? Not my time it seemed. No doubt using the toilet so much that night and copiously throwing up black tar-like gunk must have helped to eradicate most of the toxins. I wasn't proud of myself the following morning and knew that I had attempted an extreme course of action, but still felt that, if I had succeeded, it would have at least brought me solace of sorts; I would have been one less burden for others to worry about.

I was a grown man, frustrated and unable to grasp reality. All the positive elements of my life were quashed and I felt highly embarrassed at not being able to function how I once could, with no future. Was my attempt to die really such a wrong, cowardly and unforgivable act? Whatever my forlorn, depressed mind was thinking, I couldn't sink any lower than where I was now. After a precautionary visit to the hospital and some words of advice from the psychiatrist, my existence continued. I'd been pretty dumb actually, because, having just been rescued from a foreign mental health institution, which held painful images, my hari-kari episode could have easily resulted in a swift, unwanted return.

My parents watched me like hawks for weeks after, hardly ever leaving me unattended. I could understand that I'd have to regain their trust, be honest, open up if possible and explain my fears.

Being gently weaned off medication was a real relief, after what would amount to three years of solid ritualistic pill popping. My memory slowly returned, and I could once again remember what I'd done the previous week or month, rather than constantly forgetting names, dates and which food I had consumed at earlier sittings. It also enabled me to think straight, speak my mind, get an opinion across; even solving something basic like your average crossword puzzle was an achievement. This all culminated in a breakthrough of sorts but still not nearly enough to prevent my brain from always back-tracking to those vividly nasty happenings from the past. Cognitive therapy was introduced as an out patient treatment. A cookery group, exercise class and self-sustaining activities were also deployed. Even though it was satisfying to gain basic practical skills, perhaps a 'too much too soon' syndrome emerged, because, by the time the courses terminated, the bad days or moments far outweighed any upward progression.

Birthdays and Christmases were fast passing me by as occasions I couldn't enjoy nor fully get involved in. Loudness, talking, partying, my head felt like erupting some-times. To my family I probably cut a lonely, sad figure - 'Billy-no-mates', and my painted-on smile was quite conceivably bluffing nobody. In all honesty, silence represented blissfulness for me. No mouthed expressions, no judging, right? Tragically, funerals proved even more of an ordeal and, when nearest and dearest sadly died, there would always be one person missing. Me! I reproach myself at times, but gain some fragment of comfort in knowing that they had seen at least a few of my life's best highlights. It is still sickening though, when the body can seem fit and able but the subconscious is flatly refusing to cooperate.

I must have attempted all ranges of services open to me, that is, the ones that my head could facilitate. Hand on heart, out of all of these, a psychologist and a psychotherapist (whom I still benefit from to this day) come out tops. They are not patronising, are un-biased in their opinions and, of course, they have seen all these traits before, and worse, thus giving me an insight into my own idiosyncrasies and an understanding of precisely why I accommodate them. Some-body understands! I'd shout it from the rooftops if I weren't so damned inhibited. They gave, and give me now, sterling support and I will always be indebted.

So to the present, the 'here and now'. I exist in a fashion, and take each day on merit; some are bearable, some not. I've got used to my mixed-up ways, the workings and mechanics of me, and my ears are still as big as those of African elephants for listening out. I doubt I'll ever fully get over the deep-seated conviction that others are talking about me, when probably, realistically, they aren't. My strangeness, acquired from the past, has not completely vanished. In fact strong obsessive tendencies have now evolved. I always have rigid daily routines that I feel I must do, to near enough exact times. Indeed, I am forever clock-watching. It's a coping strategy of sorts as I've realised now. Tetchiness and irritability would probably swallow me up otherwise, and could therefore leave me considerably more impaired. Most friends, and old work colleagues have fallen by the wayside, which is mainly my doing, as I can't let them see this impostor. The cheery, likeable lad of bygone times replaced by this highly strung, withdrawn, antisocial, lone character living a hermit's existence. Hardly encouraging is it? A harsh portrayal of oneself but whole-heartedly true. My trust in people, especially your every day regular human being, faded many moons ago, but at least, by disassociating and living in my own company, shut away from most contacts, the deep-rooted judgemental views that I feel coming from other people cannot be heard by me and therefore don't come into question.

It's not an ideal scenario, far from it. I do not envisage that work, romance and the little taken-for-granted things will ever materialise. I'm not dying to live. Regretfully I'm living to die, just going through the motions. When my number's up, so be it. There are plenty of individuals who have had personal battles and hardships, some who only know pain and suffering from an early age. When I do eventually meet my maker I will have had thirty-odd memorable, fulfilling years; many never get that opportunity. Without my parents strong, stoic support, and I probably severely disrupted their lives, I have no clue where I might be, or what condition I might be in, either re-institutionalised, sleeping under the stars or worse.

Regrets? Of course, especially if retracing my steps back precisely to that haunting era meant that I could alter, overturn somehow the end result, I'd do it in a flash. There I was, a typical youth growing up thinking I was invincible, unbreakable, rock solid, nothing could knock me down. How emphatically ridiculously wrong had I got it! My diagnosis was deemed to be psychosis or a psychotic episode if you like, but I've never had another one since. Couldn't 'Post Traumatic Stress' from the unprecedented actions of others be more accurate? How could I possibly make all this detail up? It's a very fine margin between truth and fiction,

So, if you're in the position of being fit and

well bodily and mentally, live each day to a maximum. Take nothing for granted; you never know what's in store. If you are unlucky enough to be branded as one of the unfortunate souls with which I was included, your persona can quickly become unrecognisable. Keep the faith is the small advice I'd give.

If penning this as a kind of legacy has made people stop, take notice, re-evaluate, then I've achieved my objective. Matters to do with the mind should not be brushed aside or forgotten about. Don't jest, stare or poke fun at the seemingly obscure behaviour of some folk. Chances are it's probably something that's out of their control. Mockery and scorn only exacerbate problems, leaving them feeling more isolated and de-humanised, when all they ever want to be is accepted. You just never know when you too could be in exactly the same position. Mental heath issues can affect anyone at any given time, even the most unsuspecting. Just ask me! I'm living proof, a cog among many.

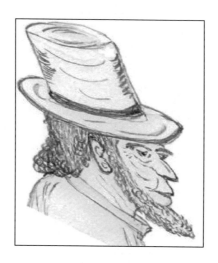

**For further information about this
or any of our publications, please
contact Martal Publications of Ipswich**

Customer Information Line 01473 720573
Email: martalbooks@msn.com

**Published and Printed
by
Martal Publications of Ipswich**
PO Box 486
IPSWICH
United Kingdom
IP4 4ZU